CLOBETASOL (PROPIONATE): A COMPREHENSIVE GUIDE

Effective Treatment Strategies for Skin Disorders

Dr. Santos Marko

Contents

CHAPTER ONE 3

Skin Infections and Causes 3

Clobetasol propionate (Clobetasol Propionate) 10

Mechanism of Action . 14

Forms and Usage of Clobetasol propionate . 15

Benefits of Using Clobetasol propionate . 21

CHAPTER TWO 24

Interactions to Avoid .. 24

Common Side Effects . 28

Alternatives to Clobetasol propionate . 31

Common Errors to Avoid 37

When to Visit a Skincare Specialist 43

THE END 49

CHAPTER ONE

Skin Infections and Causes

Skin infections involve certain physical discomforts on the skin that could be caused by bacteria, fungi, parasites, and viruses. An absolute understanding of the causes, symptoms, preventive, and treatment measures to be adopted is crucial in tackling the various skin infections experienced. Some common skin infections are impetigo, cellulitis, ringworm, athlete's foot, yeast infections, and herpes simplex virus.

Impetigo is caused by bacteria, and it is characterized by reddish sores around the nose and mouth, and sometimes hands and feet. Another bacterial causing infection of the skin is cellulitis; it is characterized by breaking, swelling, and reddening of the affected skin area.

Ringworm is a fungus causing infection of the skin that can be contacted by direct contact with an infectious fluid.

Commonly called tinea pedis, athlete's foot is a fungus-causing infection affecting the feet. It is characterized by itching of the affected area. Yeast infections are caused by the fungus, with symptoms ranging from itching, and irritations in the vaginal areas. herpes simplex virus is an infection that can be contacted through direct contact with infected fluids. Patients with such infection should seek the immediate attention of the doctor as it can only be managed, not cured.

Clobetasol propionate (Clobetasol Propionate)

Despite the high number of treatment options for

the treatment of skin infections, Clobetasol propionate comes highly recommended due to its effective nature, and minimal side effects especially when used as instructed.

It is a potent skin-applied medication for the sole purpose of treating various infections troubling the skin such as herpes, athlete's foot, yeast infections, cellulitis, impetigo, ringworm, etc.

As well as inflammations characterized by reddening, itching, and swelling of the affected skin area, which are often caused by Eczema, Psoriasis, Dermatitis, and several other inflammatory conditions of the skin.

Mechanism of Action

Clobetasol propionate works by hindering the response of the immune system and the release of inflammatory substances in the skin, hence reducing the inflammatory reactions of the skin, as well as other skin-related reactions and disorders.

Forms and Usage of Clobetasol propionate

This medication is available in different

forms, and the best formulation to apply or use would be determined by the type of skin infection, and the area of the skin infected. The Ointment form of clobetasol propionate is specially used for conditions where the skin is dry, or scaly. Its greasy form helps to soften the area of the skin upon which it is applied; aiding easy penetration of the topical applicant into the targeted area of the skin. The cream formulation is lighter, and less greasy compared to the ointment version. It is best applied on larger skin areas. The shampoo formulation is best recommended for conditions affecting the scalp regions such as psoriasis, etc. Irrespective of the formulation to be used, the dosing and length of usage of the medication should be ascertained by a skincare specialist after testing and making proper diagnosis. The formulation, application doses, and period of usage would be determined by the type of infection, severity of infection, and the area of skin infected.

Benefits of Using Clobetasol propionate

Clobetasol propionate has proven to be efficient against a number of skin-related infections such as psoriasis, eczema, dermatitis, dandruffs, ringworms, athlete's foot, cellulitis, herpes, and several other skin-related infections, and inflammatory reactions. Despite its effective nature, it is vital to consult a skincare specialist before embarking on its usage.

CHAPTER TWO

Interactions to Avoid

Interactions occur when two or more medically used topicals are used together, or during the same duration of time.

Interactions can cause either or both topically applied medications to become ineffective, whilst leaving causing disturbing side effects to the skin. Patients should avoid using clobetasol propionate along with other similar corticosteroids to avoid experiencing side effects. Always ensure to get the approval of a skincare specialist before embarking on the use of any other corticosteroid aside Clobetasol propionate.

Common Side Effects

Clobetasol propionate usage can lead to the manifestation of certain side effects especially if not adequately used.

Patients can experience skin irritations such as

itching, stinging, and burning of the application area. Using clobetasol propionate excessively and over a longer period of time can lead to skin thinning, while causing the skin to become more fragile. Other allergic reactions such as swellings, and rashes on the application areas can also be experienced.

Alternatives to Clobetasol propionate

There are numerous alternatives to consider when seeking to replace Clobetasol propionate formulations. However, these alternatives would be determined by a skincare specialist who would consider your history with skin infections, the type of infection you are currently experiencing, the region of the skin affected, the severity of the skin infection, and your tolerance to clobetasol propionate and other similar corticosteroids. Hence, do not use any other alternative to clobetasol propionate without the approval of a skincare specialist.

For less serious skin conditions, patients are advised to consider the usage of desonide. For potent topicals with lesser risks of side effects, patients should consider using betamethasone. For cases such as eczema, tacrolimus would be best recommended.

As earlier said, it is most advisable to get the approval of a skincare specialist before embarking on the usage of any alternative, so as to avoid harmful interactions that would lead to further skin complications.

Common Errors to Avoid

It is most advised to consult a skincare specialist before engaging clobetasol propionate, or any other corticosteroid. This is to ensure you are properly guided throughout the course of usage. Avoid self-medication.

Applying any of the formulations on non-affected areas of the skin can cause the applied area to itch, and become reddening.

Patients often attempt to overdose the medications to quicken the progress of the medication. This is extremely harmful and can worsen the skin infection, making the skin vulnerable to injuries in most cases.

Applying the cream formulation after properly washing and drying your hands with a clean towel is essential in preventing germs, and other infections from penetrating the affected skin during application.

Patients sometimes tend to hide these side effects out of embarrassment. Hesitating to treat these side effects can prolong the infection already experienced while adding other complications.

Always report any side effects experienced to the skincare specialist overseeing the treatment of your skin infection.

When to Visit a Skincare Specialist

Persons experiencing any symptoms of bacteria, fungus, or virus causing infections should not hesitate to call or visit a skincare specialist for urgent treatment.

It is also crucial to visit a skincare specialist whenever certain side effects are experienced during clobetasol propionate usage, a skincare specialist is best placed to make the most appropriate adjustments to the dosages of the formulations used by the patient. Endeavor to keep up with any skincare therapy session or program as instructed by a skincare specialist.

THE END

www.ingramcontent.com/pod-product-compliance
Lightning Source LLC
Chambersburg PA
CBHW072019230526
45479CB00008B/299